The Ultimate Lunch Diabetic Cookbook For The Newly Diagnosed

Easy And Delicious Lunch Diabetic Recipes

Amy Law

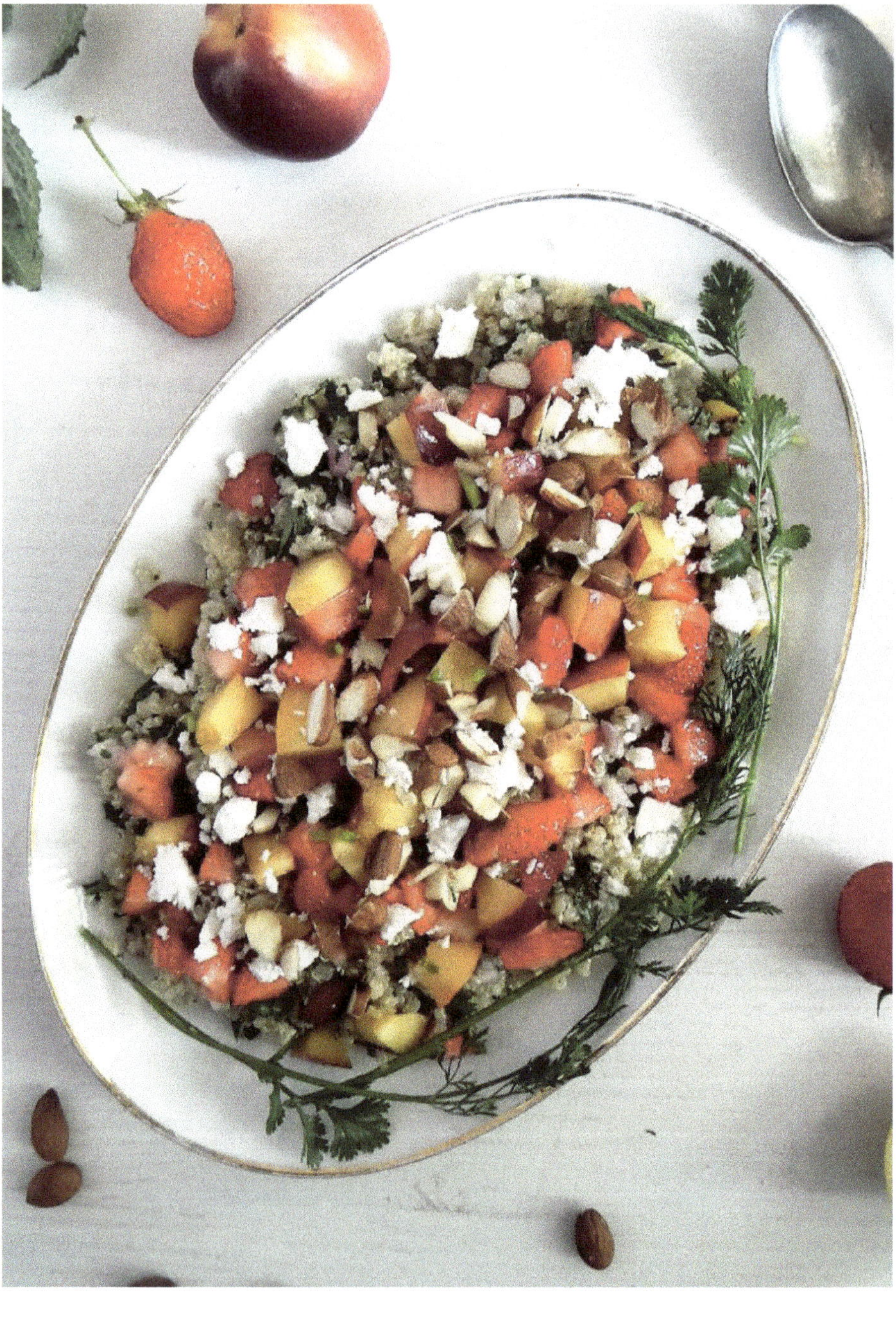

Table of contents

Chicken Tortilla Soup

Preparation Time: 10 minutes

Cooking Time: 35 minutes

Servings: 4

Ingredients:

- 1 tbsp. extra-virgin olive oil 1 onion, thinly sliced
- 1 garlic clove, minced
- jalapeño pepper, diced
- boneless, skinless chicken breasts
- 4 cups low-sodium chicken broth
- Roma tomato, diced
- ½ tsp. salt
- (6-inch) corn tortillas
- 1 lime, juiced
- Minced fresh cilantro, for garnish
- ¼ cup shredded cheddar cheese, for garnish

Direction:

1. In a medium pot, cook oil over medium-high heat. Add the onion and cook for 3 to 5 minutes until it begins to soften.

2. Add the garlic and jalapeño, and cook until fragrant, about 1minute more.
3. Add the chicken, chicken broth, tomato, and salt to the pot and boil. Lower heat to medium and simmer mildly for 20 to 25minutes.
4. Remove the chicken from the pot and set it aside.
5. Preheat a broiler to high.
6. Spray the tortilla strips with nonstick cooking spray and toss to coat. Spread in a single layer on a baking sheet and broil for 3 to 5minutes, flipping once, until crisp.
7. Once the chicken is cooked, shred it with 2 forks and return to the pot.
8. Season the soup with the lime juice. Serve hot, garnished with cilantro, cheese, and tortilla strips.

Nutrition:

Calories: 191 Carbohydrates: 13g Sugar: 2g

Beef and Mushroom Barley Soup

Preparation Time: 10 minutes

Cooking Time: 80 minutes

Servings: 6

Ingredients:

- 1 lb. beef stew meat, cubed
- ¼ tsp. salt
- ¼ tsp. freshly ground black pepper 1 tbsp. extra-virgin olive oil
- 8 oz. sliced mushrooms
- 1 onion, chopped
- carrots, chopped
- celery stalks, chopped
- 6 garlic cloves, minced
- ½ tsp. dried thyme
- cups low-sodium beef broth
- 1 cup water
- ½ cup pearl barley

Direction:

1. Season the meat well.
2. In a Pressure Pot, heat the oil over high heat. Cook meat on all sides. Remove from the pot and set aside.
3. Add the mushrooms to the pot and cook for 1 to 2 minutes. Remove the mushrooms and set them aside with the meat.
4. Sauté onion, carrots, and celery for 3 to 4 minutes. Add the garlic and continue to cook until fragrant, about 30 seconds longer.
5. Return the meat and mushrooms to the pot, then add the thyme, beef broth, and water. Adjust the pressure on high and cook for 15minutes. Let the pressure release naturally.
6. Open the Pressure Pot and add the barley. Use the slow cooker function on the Pressure Pot, affix the lid (vent open), and continue to cook for1 hour. Serve.

Nutrition:

Calories: 245 Carbohydrates: 19g Sugar: 3g

Tomato and Guaca Salad

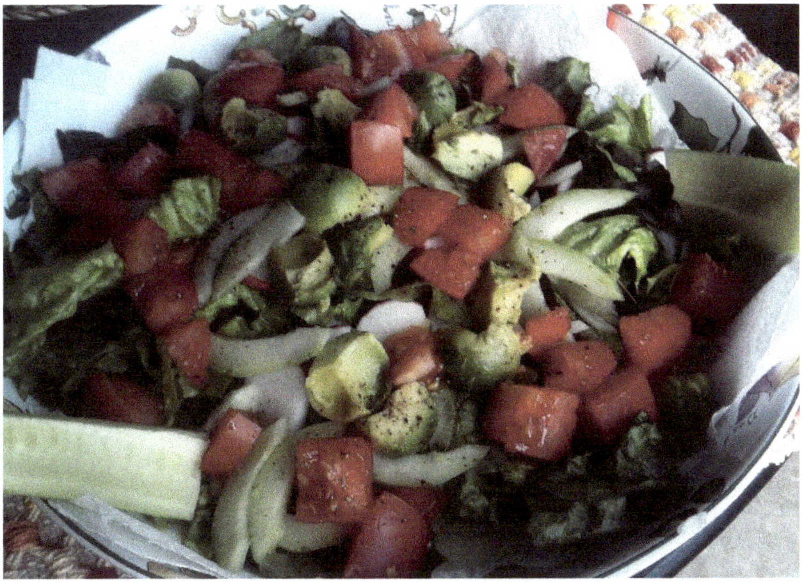

Preparation Time: 10 minutes

Cooking Time: 0 minute

Servings: 4

Ingredients:

- 1 cup cherry tomatoes
- 1 large cucumber
- 1 small red onion
- Avocado
- tbsp. chopped fresh dill

- 2 tbsp. extra-virgin olive oil
- 1 lemon, juiced
- ¼ tsp. salt
- ¼ tsp. freshly ground black pepper

Direction:

1. In a big mixing bowl, mix the tomatoes, cucumber, onion, avocado, and dill.
2. In a small bowl, combine the oil, lemon juice, salt, and pepper, and mix well.
3. Drizzle the dressing over the vegetables and toss to combine. Serve.

Nutrition:

Calories: 151 Carbohydrates: 11g Sugar: 4g

Coleslaw

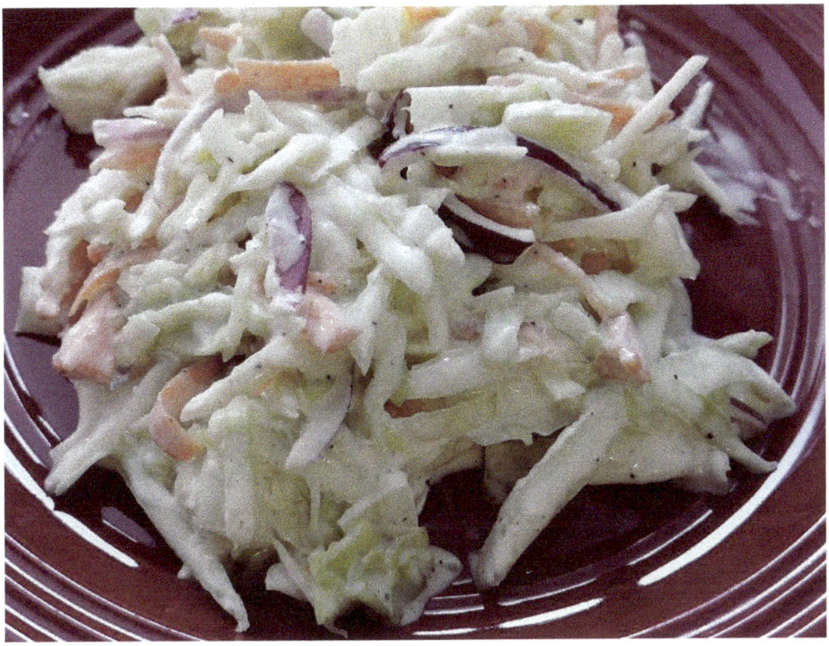

Preparation Time: 15 minutes

Cooking Time: 0 minute

Servings: 4

Ingredients:

- 2 cups green cabbage
- 2 cups red cabbage
- cups gratedcarrots
- scallions

- 2 tbsp. extra-virgin olive oil
- 2 tbsp. rice vinegar
- 1 tsp. honey
- Garlic clove
- ¼ tsp. salt

Direction:

1. Throw together the green and red cabbage, carrots, and scallions.
2. In a small bowl, whisk together the oil, vinegar, honey, garlic, and salt.
3. Pour the dressing over the veggies and mix to thoroughly combine.
4. Serve immediately, or cover and chill for several hours before serving.

Nutrition:

Calories: 80 Carbohydrates: 10g Sugar: 6g

Green Salad with Berries and Sweet Potatoes

Preparation Time: 15 minutes

Cooking Time: 20 minutes

Servings: 4

Ingredients:

For the vinaigrette:

- 1-pint blackberries
- tbsp. red wine vinegar
- 1 tbsp. honey
- tbsp. extra-virgin olive oil
- ¼ tsp. salt
- Freshly ground black pepper

For The Salad:

- 1 sweet potato, cubed
- 1 tsp. extra-virgin olive oil
- 8 cups salad greens (baby spinach, spicy greens, romaine)
- ½ red onion, sliced
- ¼ cup crumbled goat cheese

Direction:

For The Vinaigrette:

1. In a blender jar, combine the blackberries, vinegar, honey, oil, salt, and pepper, and process until smooth. Set aside.

For The Salad:

2. Preheat the oven to 425°F. Line a baking sheet with parchment paper.
3. Mix the sweet potato with the olive oil. Transfer to the prepared baking sheet and roast for 20 minutes, stirring once halfway through, until tender. Remove and cool for a few minutes.
4. In a large bowl, toss the greens with the red onion and cooled sweet potato, and drizzle with the vinaigrette.
5. Serve topped with 1 tbsp. goat cheese per serving.

Nutrition:

Calories: 196 Carbohydrates: 21g Sugar: 10g

Bean and Scallion Salad

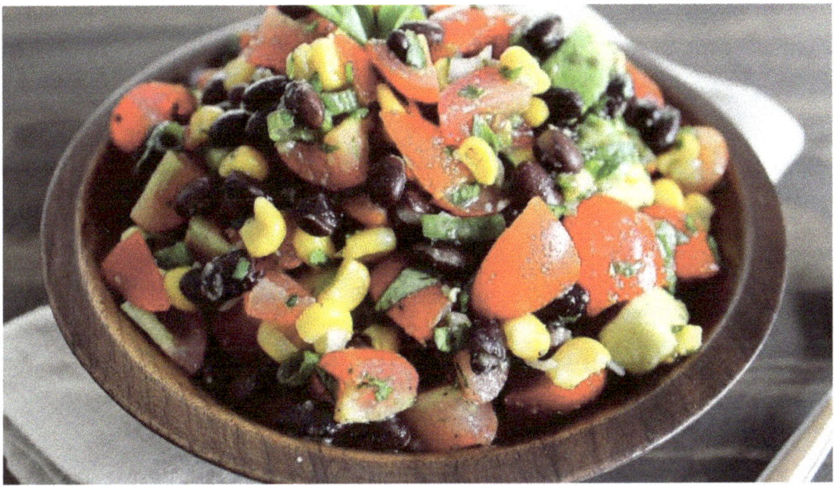

Preparation Time: 10 minutes

Cooking Time: 0 minute

Servings: 8

Ingredients:

- 1 (15 oz.) can low-sodium chickpeas
- (15 oz.) can low-sodium kidney beans
- 1 (15 oz.) can low-sodium white beans
- 1 red bell pepper
- ¼ cup chopped scallions
- ¼ cup finely chopped fresh basil

- 3 garlic cloves, minced
- tbsp. extra-virgin olive oil
- 1 tbsp. red wine vinegar
- 1 tsp. Dijon mustard
- ¼ tsp. freshly ground black pepper

Direction:

1. Toss chickpeas, kidney beans, white beans, bell pepper, scallions, basil, and garlic gently.
2. Blend together olive oil, vinegar, mustard, and pepper. Toss with the salad.
3. Wrap and chill for 1hour.

Nutrition:

Calories: 193 Carbohydrates: 29g Sugar: 3g

Rainbow Bean Salad

Preparation Time: 15 minutes

Cooking Time: 0 minute

Servings: 5

Ingredients:

- 1 (15 oz.) can low-sodium black beans
- 1 avocado, diced
- 1 cup cherry
- 3 tomatoes, halved
- 1 cup chopped baby spinach
- ½ cup red bell pepper
- ¼ cup jicama
- ½ cup scallions
- ¼ cup fresh cilantro
- 2 tbsp. lime juice
- 1 tbsp. extra-virgin olive oil
- 2 garlic cloves, minced
- 1 tsp. honey
- ¼ tsp. salt
- ¼ tsp. freshly ground black pepper

Direction:

1. Mix black beans, avocado, tomatoes, spinach, bell pepper, jicama, scallions, and cilantro.
2. Blend lime juice, oil, garlic, honey, salt, and pepper. Add to the salad and toss.
3. Chill for 1 hour before serving.

Nutrition:

Calories: 169 Carbohydrates: 22g Sugar: 3g

Warm Barley and Squash Salad

Preparation Time: 20 minutes

Cooking Time: 40 minutes

Servings: 8

Ingredients:

- 1 small butternut squash
- 3 tbsp. extra-virgin olive oil
- 2 cups broccoli florets
- 1 cup pearl barley
- cup toasted chopped walnuts
- 2 cups baby kale
- ½ red onion, sliced
- tbsp. balsamic vinegar
- 2 garlic cloves, minced
- ½ tsp. salt
- ¼ tsp. black pepper

Direction:

1. Preheat the oven to 400°F. Line a baking sheet with parchment paper.

2. Peel off the squash, and slice into dice. In a large bowl, toss the squash with 2 tsp. of olive oil. Transfer to the prepared baking sheet and roast for 20minutes.
3. While the squash is roasting, toss the broccoli in the same bowl with 1 tsp. of olive oil. After 20 minutes, flip the squash and push it to one side of the baking sheet. Add the broccoli to the other side and continue to roast for 20 more minutes until tender.
4. While the veggies are roasting, in a medium pot, cover the barley with several inches of water. Boil, then adjust heat, cover, and simmer for30 minutes until tender. Drain and rinse.
5. Transfer the barley to a large bowl, and toss with the cooked squash and broccoli, walnuts, kale, and onion.
6. In a small bowl, mix the remaining 2 tbsp. olive oil, balsamic vinegar, garlic, salt, and pepper. Drizzle dressing over the salad and toss.

Nutrition:

Calories: 274 Carbohydrates: 32g Sugar: 3g

Citrus and Chicken Salad

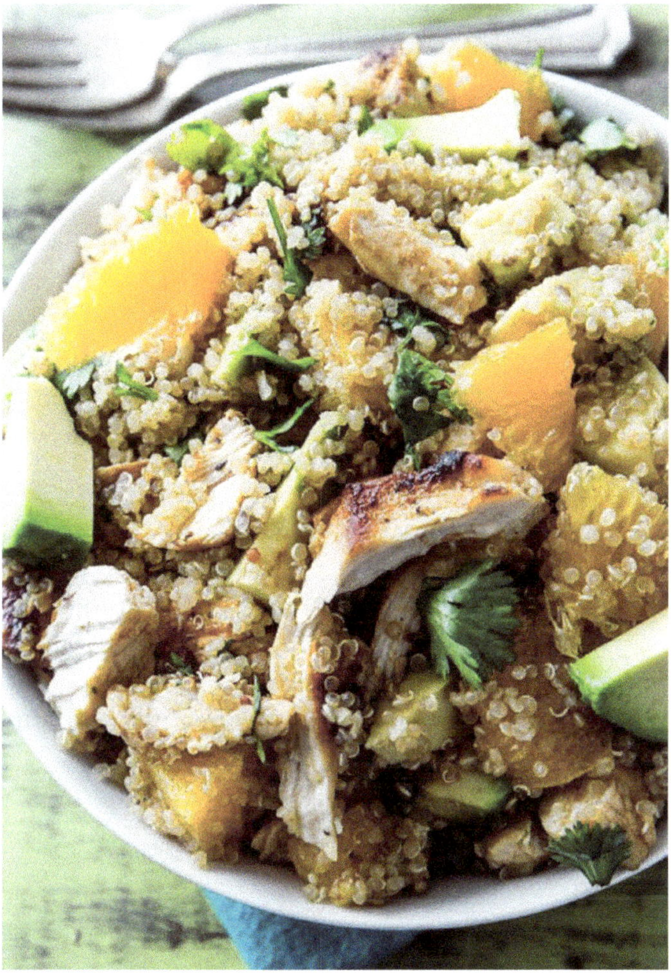

Preparation Time: 10 minutes

Cooking Time: 0 minute

Servings: 4

Ingredients:

- 4 cups baby spinach
- 2 tbsp. extra-virgin olive oil
- 1 tbsp. lemon juice
- ⅛ tsp. salt
- 2 cups chopped cooked chicken
- 2 mandarin oranges
- ½ peeled grapefruit, sectioned
- ¼ cup sliced almonds

Direction:

1. Toss spinach with the olive oil, lemon juice, salt, and pepper.
2. Add the chicken, oranges, grapefruit, and almonds to the bowl. Toss gently.
3. Arrange on 4 plates and serve.

Nutrition:

Calories: 249 Carbohydrates: 11g Sugar: 7g

Blueberry and Chicken Salad

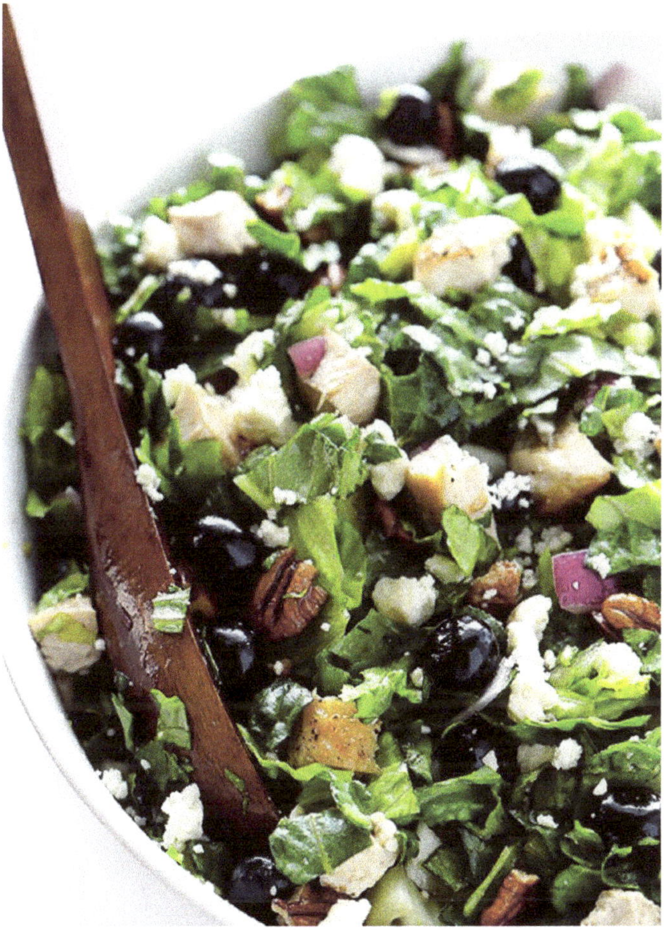

Preparation Time: 10 minutes

Cooking Time: 0 minute

Servings: 4

Ingredients:

- 2 cups chopped cooked chicken
- 1 cup fresh blueberries
- ¼ cup almonds 1 celery stalk
- ¼ cup red onion
- 1 tbsp. fresh basil
- 1 tbsp. fresh cilantro
- ½ cup plain, vegan mayonnaise
- ¼ tsp. salt
- ¼ tsp. freshly ground black pepper
- 8 cups salad greens

Direction:

1. Toss chicken, blueberries, almonds, celery, onion, basil, and cilantro.
2. Blend yogurt, salt, and pepper. Stir chicken salad to combine.
3. Situate 2 cups of salad greens on each of 4 plates and divide the chicken salad among the plates to serve.

Nutrition:

Calories: 207 Carbohydrates: 11g Sugar: 6g

Crunchy Strawberry Salad

Preparation Time: 10 minutes

Cooking Time: 0 minutes

Servings: 5

Ingredients:

- 0.6 lb. romaine lettuce leaves, roughly torn
- 0.6 lb. strawberries, sliced
- 0.2 lb. nuts of choice

Directions:

1. In a large mixing bowl add strawberry slices, lettuce, and nuts; toss to combine.
2. Add to a serving bowl.

Nutrition:

Calories: 94 Fat: 0.3g Protein: 11g

Zucchini Noodle Salad with Almonds

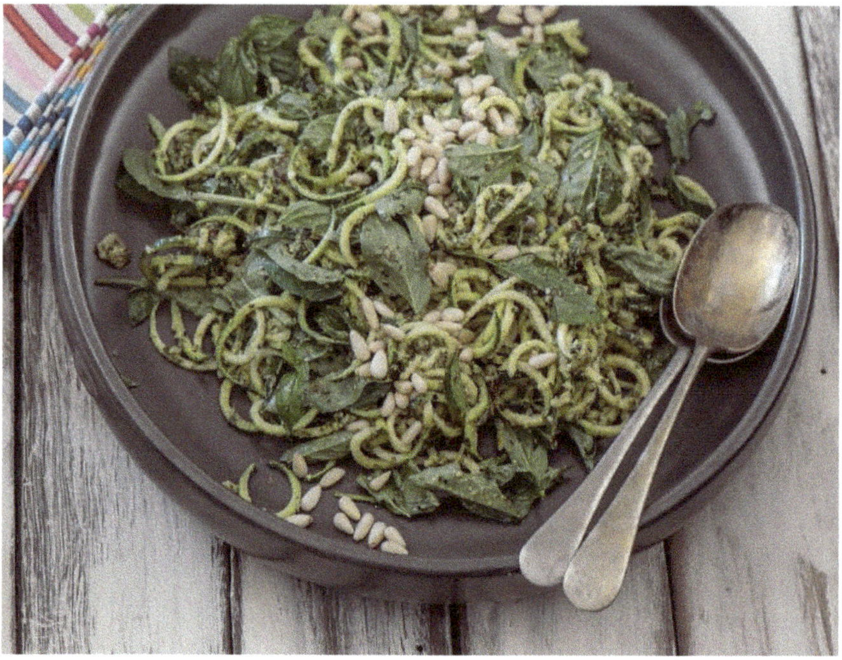

Preparation Time: 35 minutes

Cooking Time: 10 minutes

Servings: 4

Ingredients:

- 2–3 zucchini, noodle
- 2 tbsp. olive oil
- 1 carrot, peeled, noodled
- lb. red cabbage, thinly sliced

- 2 tbsp. lime juice
- Kosher salt and pepper, to taste
- lb. toasted almonds, chopped
- 3–4 tbsp. cilantro leaves

Directions:

1. Combine zucchini, carrots, cabbage, and almonds. Season with salt, pepper, lemon juice, and olive oil then toss it well.
2. Add to a serving platter.

Nutrition:

Calories: 264 Fat: 2g Protein: 6g

Carrot and Spinach Salad

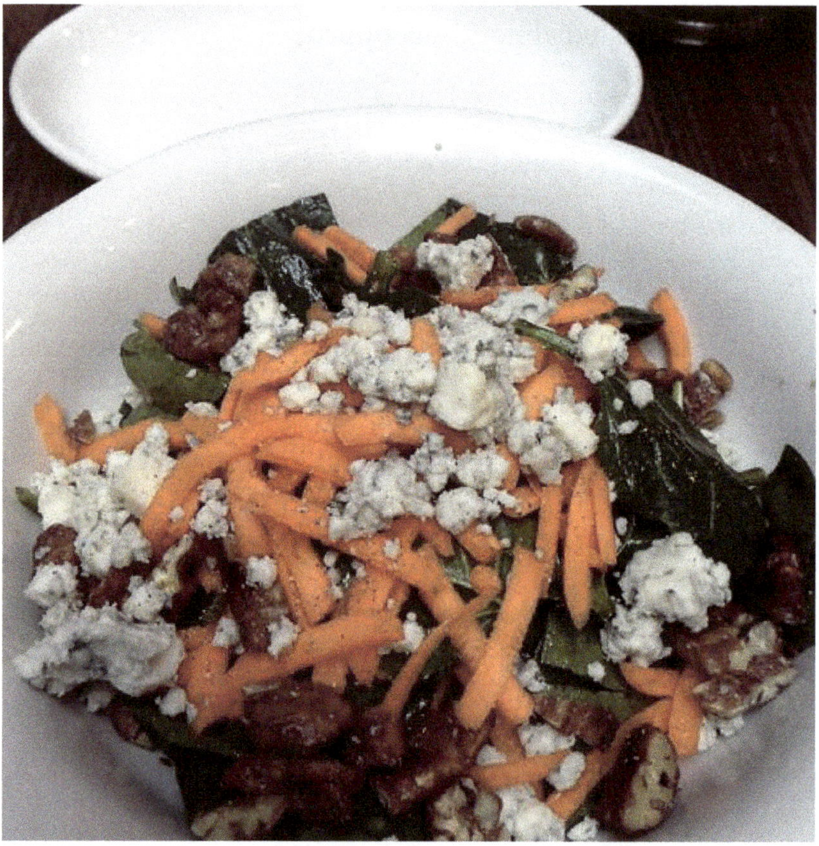

Preparation Time: 60 minutes

Cooking Time: 0 minutes

Servings: 4

Ingredients:

- 0.8 lb. baby spinach leaves

- 2 carrots, peeled, grated
- 5 tbsp. olive oil
- 4 tbsp. lemon juice
- Salt and black pepper, to taste
- 1 tsp. thyme
- 1–2 garlic cloves, minced
- ¼ tsp. olive powder

Directions:

1. Stir in lemon juice, olive oil, salt, pepper, onion powder, and garlic. Mix well.
2. Add carrots and spinach leaves to the mixture. Toss to combine.
3. Cover the bowl with a plastic wrapper. Place it in the refrigerator for about 50 minutes before serving.

Nutrition:

Calories: 215 Fat: 4.5g Protein: 14g

Red Cabbage Salad

Preparation Time: 15 minutes

Cooking Time: 0 minutes

Servings: 4

Ingredients:

- lb. red cabbage, thinly sliced
- 2 carrots, peeled, thinly sliced
- 2 tbsp. olive oil
- Salt and black pepper, to taste
- 2 tbsp. lemon juice
- tbsp. coriander leaves,c hopped
- 1 tbsp. mint leaves, chopped

Directions:

Combine cabbage, carrots, mint, and coriander. Mix in salt, pepper, lemon juice, and olive oil then toss it well. Transfer salad onto a serving platter.

Nutrition:

Calories: 226 Fat: 5g Protein: 12g

Quinoa Fruit Salad

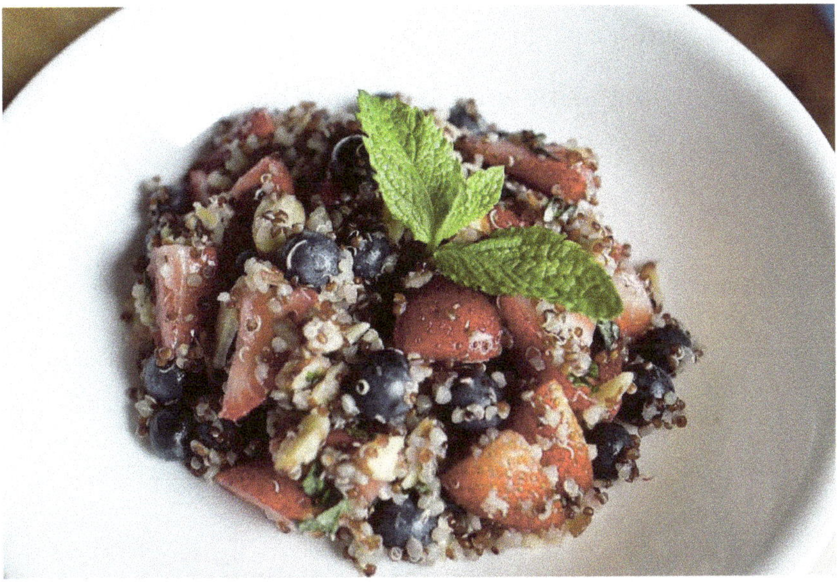

Preparation Time: 15 minutes

Cooking Time: 0 minutes

Servings: 3

Ingredients:

- 1 lb. cooked quinoa
- 1 mango, peeled and diced
- ½ lb. strawberries, quartered
- ½ lb. blueberries
- 2 tbsp. pine nuts

- Chopped mint leaves, for garnish
- 4 tbsp. olive oil
- 1 lemon zest, as required
- 3 tbsp. freshly squeezed lemon juice
- 1 tbsp. date sugar

Directions:

1. For the vinaigrette, beat the olive oil, lemon zest, juice, and sugar in a small bowl. Set aside.
2. Mix quinoa, mango, strawberries, blueberries, and pine nuts in a large bowl.
3. Add the lemon vinaigrette.

Nutrition:

Calories: 490 Fat: 17.2g Protein: 9.8g

Beef and Red Bean Chili

Preparation Time: 10 minutes

Cooking Time: 6 hours

Servings: 4

Ingredients:

- cup dry red beans 1 tbsp. olive oil
- pounds' boneless beef chuck
- large onion, coarsely chopped
- 1 (14 ounces) can beef broth
- chipotle chili peppers in adobo sauce
- 2 tsp. dried oregano, crushed
- 1 tsp. ground cumin
- ½ tsp. salt
- 1 (14.5 ounces) can tomatoes with mild green chilis
- 1 (15 ounces) can tomato sauce
- ¼ cup snipped fresh cilantro
- 1 medium red sweet pepper

Direction:

1. Rinse out the beans and place them into a Dutch oven or big saucepan, then add in water enough to cover them. Allow the beans to boil then drop the heat down. Simmer the beans without a cover for 10 minutes. Take off the heat and keep covered for an hour.
2. In a big frypan, heat up the oil upon medium-high heat, then cook onion and half the beef until they brown a bit over medium-high heat. Move into a 3 ½ or 4-quart crockery cooker. Do this again with what's left of the beef. Add in tomato sauce, tomatoes (not drained), salt, cumin, oregano, adobo sauce, chipotle peppers, and broth, stirring to blend. Strain out and rinse beans and stir in the cooker.
3. Cook while covered on a low setting for around 10–12 hours or on a high setting for 5–6 hours. Spoon the chili into bowls or mugs and top with sweet pepper and cilantro.

Nutrition:

Calories: 288 Carbohydrate: 24g Sugar: 5g

Berry Apple Cider

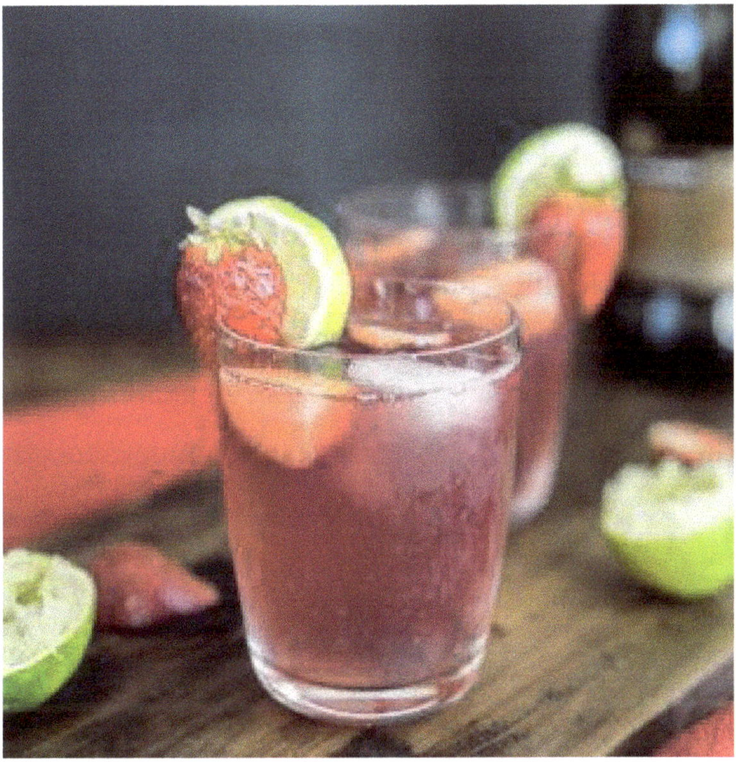

Preparation Time: 15 minutes

Cooking Time: 3 hours

Servings: 3

Ingredients:

- 4 cinnamon sticks, cut into 1-inch pieces
- 1½ tsp. whole cloves

- 4 cups apple cider
- 4 cups low-calorie cranberry-raspberry juice drink
- 1 medium apple

Direction:

1. To make the spice bag, cut out a 6-inch square from double-thick, pure cotton cheesecloth. Put in the cloves and cinnamon, then bring the corners up, tie it closed using a clean kitchen string that is pure cotton.
2. In a 3 ½ 5-quart slow cooker, combine cranberry-raspberry juice, apple cider, and the spice bag.
3. Cook while covered over a low heat setting for around 4–6 hours or on a high heat setting for 2-2 ½hours.
4. Throw out the spice bag. Serve right away or keep it warm while covered on warm or low-heat setting up to 2 hours, occasionally stirring. Garnish each serving with apples (thinly sliced).

Nutrition:

Calories: 89 Carbohydrate: 22g Sugar: 19g

Brunswick Stew

Preparation Time: 10 minutes

Cooking Time: 45 minutes

Servings: 3

Ingredients:

- 4 oz. diced salt pork
- pounds' chicken parts
- 8 cupswater
- 3 potatoes,cubed
- 3 onions, chopped
- 1 (28 oz.) can whole peeled tomatoes
- 2 cups canned whole kernel corn
- 1 (10 oz.) package frozen lima beans
- 1 tbsp. Worcestershire sauce
- ½ tsp. salt
- ¼ tsp. ground black pepper

Direction:

1. Mix and boil water, chicken, and salt pork in a big pot on high heat. Lower heat to low. Cover then simmer until chicken is tender for45 minutes.

2. Take out chicken. Let cool until easily handled. Take the meat out. Throw out bones and skin. Chop meat into bite-sized pieces. Put back in the soup.
3. Add ground black pepper, salt, Worcestershire sauce, lima beans, corn, tomatoes, onions, and potatoes. Mix well. Stir well and simmer for 1 hour, uncovered.

Nutrition:

Calories: 368 Carbohydrate: 25.9g Protein: 27.9g

Buffalo Chicken Salads

Preparation Time: 7 minutes

Cooking Time: 3 hours

Servings: 5

Ingredients:

- 1½ pounds chicken breast halves
- ½ cup Wing Time Buffalo chicken sauce
- 4 tsp. cider vinegar
- tsp. Worcestershire sauce
- 1 tsp. paprika
- 1/3 cup light mayonnaise
- 2 tbsp. fat-free milk
- tbsp. crumbled blue cheese
- 2 romaine hearts, chopped
- cup whole-grain croutons
- ½ cup very thinly sliced red onion

Direction:

1. Place chicken in a 2/4 slow cooker. Mix together Worcestershire sauce, 2 tsp. of vinegar and Buffalo sauce in a small bowl; pour over chicken. Dust with

paprika. Close and cook for 3 hours on a low-heat setting.

2. Mix the leftover 2 tsp. of vinegar with milk and light mayonnaise together in a small bowl at serving time; mix in blue cheese. While chicken is still in the slow cooker, pull meat into bite-sized pieces using 2forks.
3. Split the romaine among 6 dishes. Spoon sauce and chicken over lettuce. Pour with blue cheese dressing then add red onion slices and croutons on top.

Nutrition:

Calories: 274 Carbohydrate: 11g Fiber: 2g

Cacciatore Style Chicken

Preparation Time: 10 minutes

Cooking Time: 4 hours

Servings: 6

Ingredients:

- cups sliced fresh mushrooms
- 1 cup sliced celery
- cup chopped carrot
- medium onions, cut into wedges
- 1 green, yellow, or red sweet peppers
- 4 garlic cloves, minced
- 12 chicken drumsticks
- ½ cup chicken broth
- ¼ cup dry white wine
- 2 tbsp. quick-cooking tapioca
- 2 bay leaves
- 1 tsp. dried oregano, crushed
- 1 tsp. sugar
- ½ tsp. salt
- ¼ tsp. pepper
- 1 (14.5 ounces) can diced tomatoes

- 1/3 cup tomato paste Hot cooked pasta or rice

Direction:

1. Mix garlic, sweet pepper, onions, carrot, celery, and mushrooms in a 5 or 6-qt. slow cooker. Cover veggies with the chicken. Add pepper, salt, sugar, oregano, bay leaves, tapioca, wine, and broth.
2. Cover. Cook for 3–3 ½ hours on a high-heat setting.
3. Take chicken out; keep warm. Discard bay leaves. Turn to the high- heat setting if using the low-heat setting. Mix tomato paste and undrained tomatoes in. Cover. Cook on high-heat setting for 15 more minutes.
4. Servings**:** Put the veggie mixture on top of pasta and chicken.

Nutrition:

Calories: 324 Sugar: 7g Carbohydrates: 35g

Carnitas Tacos

Preparation Time: 10 minutes

Cooking Time: 5 hours

Servings: 4

Ingredients:

- 3 to 3½ lb. bone-in pork shoulder roast
- ½ cup chopped onion
- 1/3 cup orange juice
- 1 tbsp. ground cumin
- 1½ tsp. kosher salt
- tsp. dried oregano, crushed
- ¼ tsp. cayenne pepper
- 1 lime
- (5.3 ounces) containers plain low-fat Greek yogurt
- 1 pinch kosher salt
- 16 (6 inches) soft yellow corn tortillas
- 4 leaves green cabbage, quartered
- 1 cup very thinly sliced red onion
- 1 cup salsa (optional)

Direction:

1. Take off meat from the bone; throw away bone. Trim meat fat. Slice meat into 2 to 3-inch pieces; put in a slow cooker of 3 ½ or 4-quartin size. Mix in cayenne, oregano, salt, cumin, orange juice, and onion.
2. Cover and cook for 4 to 5 hours on high. Take out the meat from the cooker. Shred meat with 2 forks. Mix in enough cooking liquid to moisten.
3. Take out 1 tsp. zest (put aside) for lime crema, then squeeze 2tbsp. lime juice. Mix dash salt, yogurt, and lime juice in a small bowl.
4. Serve lime crema, salsa (if wished), red onion, and cabbage with meat in tortillas. Scatter with lime zest.

Nutrition:

Calories: 301 Carbohydrate: 28g Sugar: 7g

Chicken Vera Cruz

Preparation Time: 7 minutes

Cooking Time: 10 hours

Servings: 5

Ingredients:

- 1 medium onion, cut into wedges
- 1 lb. yellow-skin potatoes
- 6 skinless, boneless chicken thighs
- 2 (14.5 oz.) cans no-salt-added diced tomatoes
- 1 fresh jalapeño chili pepper
- 2 tbsp. Worcestershire sauce
- 1 tbsp. chopped garlic
- tsp. dried oregano, crushed
- ¼ tsp. ground cinnamon
- ⅛ tsp. ground cloves
- ½ cup snipped fresh parsley
- ¼ cup chopped pimiento-stuffed green olives

Direction:

1. Put the onion in a 3 ½ or 4-quart slow cooker. Place chicken thigh sand potatoes on top. Drain and discard juices from a can of tomatoes. Stir undrained and drained tomatoes, cloves, cinnamon, oregano, garlic, Worcestershire sauce, and jalapeño pepper together in a bowl. Pour over all in the cooker.
2. Cook with a cover for 10 hours on a low-heat setting.
3. To make the topping: Stir chopped pimiento-stuffed green olives and snipped fresh parsley together in a small bowl. Drizzle the topping over each serving of chicken.

Nutrition:

Calories: 228 Sugar: 9g Carbohydrate: 25g

Chicken and Cornmeal Dumplings

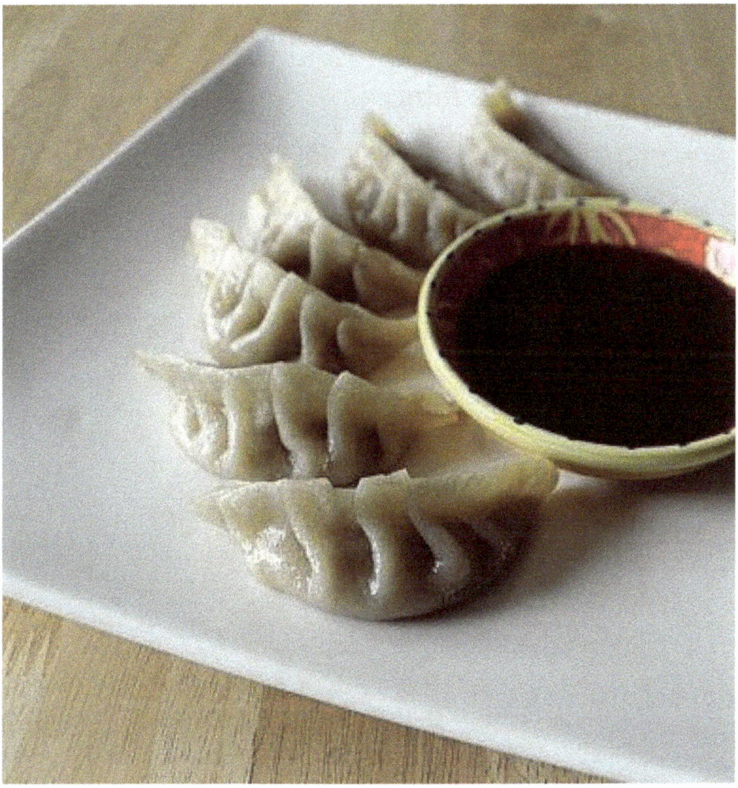

Preparation Time: 8 minutes

Cooking Time: 8 hours

Servings: 4

Ingredients:

Chicken and Vegetable Filling:

- medium carrots, thinly sliced

- 1 stalk celery, thinly sliced
- 1/3 cup corn kernels
- ½ a medium onion, thinly sliced
- 2 garlic cloves, minced
- 1 tsp. snipped fresh rosemary
- ¼ tsp. ground black pepper
- 2 chicken thighs, skinned
- 1 cup reduced-sodium chicken broth
- ½ cup fat-free milk
- 1 tbsp. all-purpose flour Corn meal

Dumplings:

- ¼ cup flour
- ¼ cup cornmeal
- ½ tsp. baking powder
- 1 egg white
- 1 tbsp. fat-free milk
- 1 tbsp. canola oil

Direction:

1. Mix ¼ tsp. pepper, carrots, garlic, celery, rosemary, corn, and onion in a 1 ½ or 2-quart slow cooker. Place chicken on top. Pour the broth atop the mixture into the cooker.

2. Close and cook on low-heat for 7 to 8hours.
3. If cooking with the low-heat setting, switch to a high-heat setting (or if the heat setting is not available, continue to cook). Place the chicken onto a cutting board and let cool slightly. Once cool enough to handle, chop off the chicken from bones and get rid of the bones. Chop the chicken and place it back into the mixture in the cooker. Mix flour and milk in a small bowl until smooth. Stir into the mixture in the cooker.
4. Drop the Cornmeal Dumplings dough into 4 mounds atop hot chicken mixture using 2 spoons. Cover and cook for 20 to 25 minutes more or until a toothpick comes out clean when inserted into a dumpling. (Avoid lifting the lid when cooking.) Sprinkle each of the serving with coarse pepper if desired.
5. Mix together ½ tsp. baking powder, ¼ cup flour, a dash of salt and, ¼ cup cornmeal in a medium bowl. Mix 1 tbsp. canola oil, 1 egg white, and 1 tbsp. fat-free milk in a small bowl. Pour the egg mixture into the flour mixture. Mix just until moistened.

Nutrition:

Calories: 369 Sugar: 9g Carbohydrates: 47g

Chicken and Pepperoni

Preparation Time: 4 minutes

Cooking Time: 4 hours

Servings: 5

Ingredients:

- 3 ½ to 4 pounds' meaty chicken pieces
- ⅛ tsp. salt
- ⅛ tsp. black pepper
- 2 oz. sliced turkey pepperoni
- ¼ cup sliced pitted ripe olives
- ½ cup reduced-sodium chicken broth
- 1 tbsp. tomato paste
- 1 tsp. dried Italian seasoning, crushed
- ½ cup shredded part-skim mozzarella cheese (2 oz.)

Direction:

1. Put the chicken into a 3 ½ to 5-qt. slow cooker. Sprinkle pepper and salt on the chicken. Slice pepperoni slices in half. Put olives and pepperoni into the slow cooker. In a small bowl, blend Italian

seasoning, tomato paste, and chicken broth together. Transfer the mixture into the slow cooker.

2. Cook with a cover for 3–3 ½ hours on high.
3. Transfer the olives, pepperoni, and chicken onto a serving platter with a slotted spoon. Discard the cooking liquid. Sprinkle cheese over the chicken. Use foil to loosely cover and allow to sit for 5 minutes to melt the cheese.

Nutrition:

Calories: 243 Carbohydrate: 1g Protein: 41g

Chicken and Sausage Gumbo

Preparation Time: 6 minutes

Cooking Time: 4 hours

Servings: 5

Ingredients:

- 1/3 cup all-purpose flour
- 1 (14 oz.) can reduced-sodium chicken broth
- 2 cups chicken breast
- 8 oz. smoked turkey sausage links
- 2 cups sliced fresh okra
- 1 cup water
- 1 cup coarsely chopped onion
- 1 cup sweet pepper
- ½ cup sliced celery
- 4 garlic cloves, minced 1 tsp. dried thyme
- ½ tsp. ground black pepper
- ¼ tsp. cayenne pepper
- 3 cups hot cooked brown rice

Direction:

1. To make the roux: Cook the flour upon medium heat in a heavy medium-sized saucepan, stirring periodically, for roughly 6 minutes or until the flour browns. Take off the heat and slightly cool, then slowly stir in the broth. Cook the roux until it bubbles and thicken sup.
2. Pour the roux in a 3 ½ or 4/4 slow cooker, then add in cayenne pepper, black pepper, thyme, garlic, celery, sweet pepper, onion, water, okra, sausage, and chicken.
3. Cook the soup covered on a high setting for 3–3 ½ hours. Take the fat off the top and serve atop hot cooked brown rice.

Nutrition:

Calories: 230 Sugar: 3g Protein: 19g

Chicken, Barley, and Leek Stew

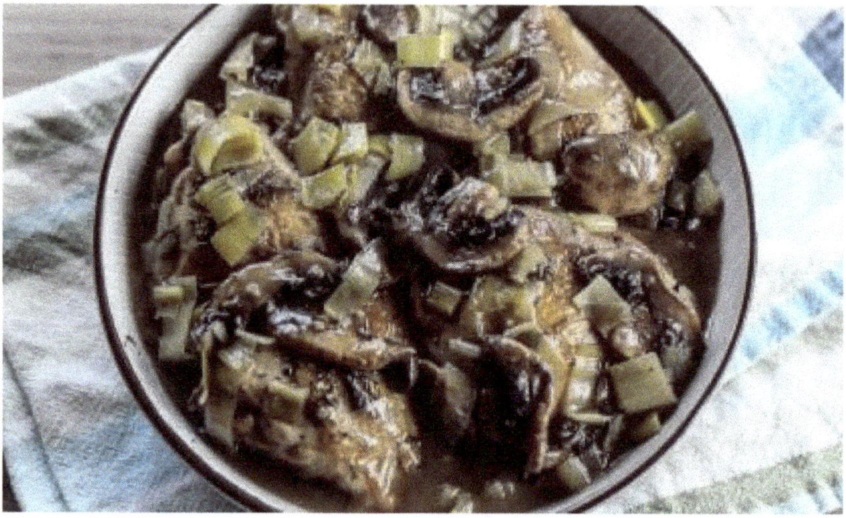

Preparation Time: 10 minutes

Cooking Time: 3 hours

Servings: 2

Ingredients:

- 1 lb. chicken thighs
- 1 tbsp. olive oil
- 1 (49 ounces) can reduced-sodium chicken broth
- cup regular barley (not quick-cooking)
- medium leeks, halved lengthwise and sliced
- 2 medium carrots, thinly sliced

- 1½ tsp. dried basil or Italian seasoning, crushed
- ¼ tsp. cracked black pepper

Direction:

1. In the big skillet, cook the chicken in hot oil till becoming brown on all sides. In the 4–5-qt. slow cooker, whisk the pepper, dried basil, carrots, leeks, barley, chicken broth, and chicken.
2. Keep covered and cooked over a high heat setting for 2–2.5 hours or till the barley softens. As you wish, drizzle with the parsley or fresh basil prior to serving.

Nutrition:

Calories: 248 Fiber: 6g Carbohydrate: 27g

Cider Pork Stew

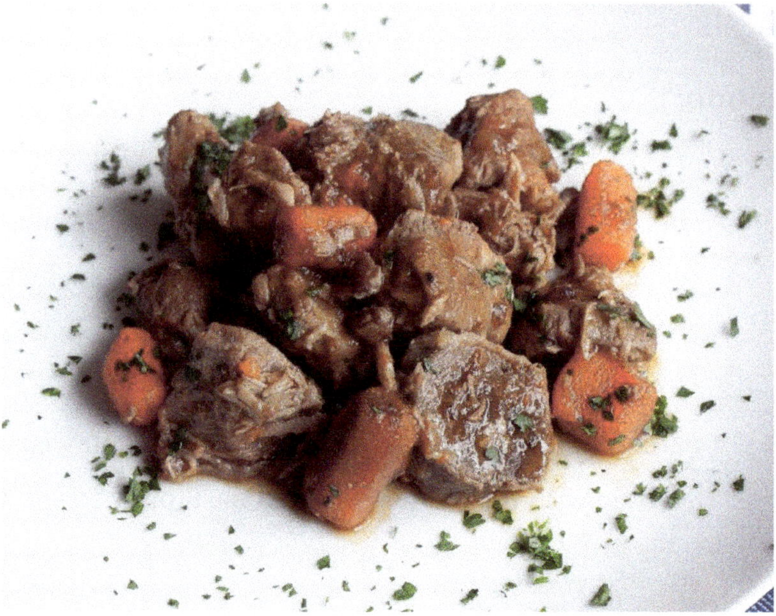

Preparation Time: 9 minutes

Cooking Time: 12 hours

Servings: 3

Ingredients:

- pounds' pork shoulder roast
- 3 medium cubed potatoes
- Medium carrots
- 2 medium onions, sliced

- 1 cup coarsely chopped apple
- ½ cup coarsely chopped celery
- 3 tbsp. quick-cooking tapioca
- 2 cups apple juice
- 1 tsp. salt
- 1 tsp. caraway seeds
- ¼ tsp. black pepper

Direction:

1. Chop the meat into 1-in. cubes. In the 3.5–5.5 qt. slow cooker, mix the tapioca, celery, apple, onions, carrots, potatoes, and meat. Whisk in pepper, caraway seeds, salt, and apple juice.
2. Keep covered and cook over a low heat setting for 10–12 hours. If you want, use the celery leaves to decorate each of the servings.

Nutrition:

Calories: 244 Fiber: 5g Carbohydrate: 33g

Creamy Chicken Noodle Soup

Preparation Time: 7 minutes

Cooking Time: 8 hours

Servings: 4

Ingredients:

- 1 (32 fluid ounce) container reduced-sodium chicken broth
- 3 cups water
- 2½ cups chopped cooked chicken
- 3 medium carrots, sliced
- 3 stalks celery
- 1½ cups sliced fresh mushrooms
- ¼ cup chopped onion
- 1½ tsp. dried thyme, crushed
- ¾ tsp. garlic-pepper seasoning
- 3 oz. reduced-fat cream cheese (Neufchâtel), cut up
- 2 cups dried egg noodles

Direction:

1. Mix together the garlic-pepper seasoning, thyme, onion, mushrooms, celery, carrots, chicken, water, and broth in a 5 to 6-quart slow cooker.
2. Put the cover and let it cook for 6–8 hours on a low-heat setting.
3. Increase to the high-heat setting if you are using a low-heat setting. Mix in the cream cheese until blended. Mix in uncooked noodles. Put the cover and let it cook for an additional 20–30 minutes or just until the noodles become tender.

Nutrition:

Calories: 170 Sugar: 3g Fiber: 2g

Cuban Pulled Pork Sandwich

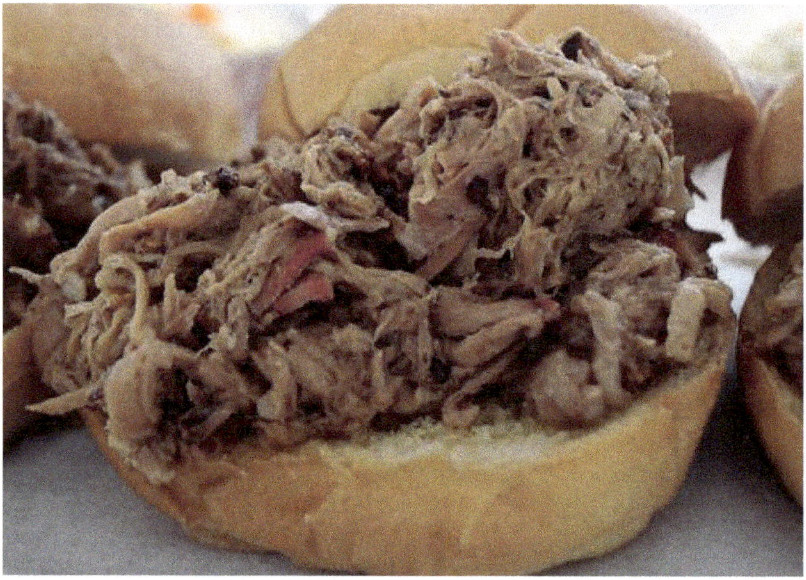

Preparation Time: 6 minutes

Cooking Time: 5 hours

Servings: 5

Ingredients:

- tsp. dried oregano, crushed
- ¾ tsp. ground cumin
- ½ tsp. ground coriander
- ¼ tsp. salt
- ¼ tsp. black pepper

- ¼ tsp. ground allspice
- 2½ lb. boneless pork shoulder roast
- 1 tbsp. olive oil
- Nonstick cooking spray
- 2 cups sliced onions
- 2 green sweet peppers, cut into bite-size strips
- ½ to 1 fresh jalapeño pepper
- 4 garlic cloves, minced
- ¼ cup orange juice
- ¼ cup lime juice
- 6 heart-healthy wheat hamburger buns, toasted
- 2 tbsp. jalapeño mustard

Direction:

1. Mix allspice, oregano, black pepper, cumin, salt, and coriander together in a small bowl. Press each side of the roast into the spice mixture. On medium-high heat, heat oil in a big non-stick pan; put in roast. Cook for 5 mins until both sides of the roast are light brown, turn the roast 1time.
2. Using a cooking spray, grease a 3 ½ or 4qt slow cooker; arrange the garlic, onions, jalapeno, and green peppers in a layer. Pour in lime juice and orange juice. Slice the roast if needed to fit inside the

cooker; put on top of the vegetables covered for 4 ½–5 hrs on high heat setting.

3. Move roast to a cutting board using a slotted spoon. Drain the cooking liquid and keep the jalapeno, green peppers, and onions. Shred the roast with 2 forks then place it back in the cooker. Remove fat from the
4. liquid. Mix half cup cooking liquid and reserved vegetables into the cooker. Pour in more cooking liquid if desired. Discard the remaining cooking liquid.
5. Slather mustard on rolls. Split the meat between the bottom roll halves. Add avocado on top if desired. Place the roll tops on sandwiches.

Nutrition:

Calories: 379 Carbohydrate: 32g Fiber: 4g

Lemon-Tarragon Soup

Preparation Time: 10 minutes

Cooking Time: 10 minutes

Servings: 2

Ingredients:

- 1 tbsp. avocado oil
- ½ cup diced onion
- 3 garlic cloves, crushed
- ¼ plus ⅛ tsp. sea salt
- ¼ plus ⅛ tsp. freshly ground black pepper
- 1 (13.5 oz.) can full-fat coconut milk
- tbsp. freshly squeezed lemon juice
- ½ cup raw cashews
- 1 celery stalk
- tbsp. chopped fresh tarragon

Directions:

1. In a medium skillet over medium-high heat, heat up avocado oil. Sauté onion, garlic, salt, and pepper for 4minutes.

2. In a high-speed blender, blend together the coconut milk, lemon juice, cashews, celery, and tarragon with the onion mixture until smooth. Adjust seasonings, if necessary.
3. Pour into 1 large or 2 small bowls and enjoy immediately, or transfer to a medium saucepan and warm on low heat for 3 to 5 minutes before serving.

Nutrition:

Calories: 264 Fiber: 11g Fats: 10g

Chilled Cucumber and Lime Soup

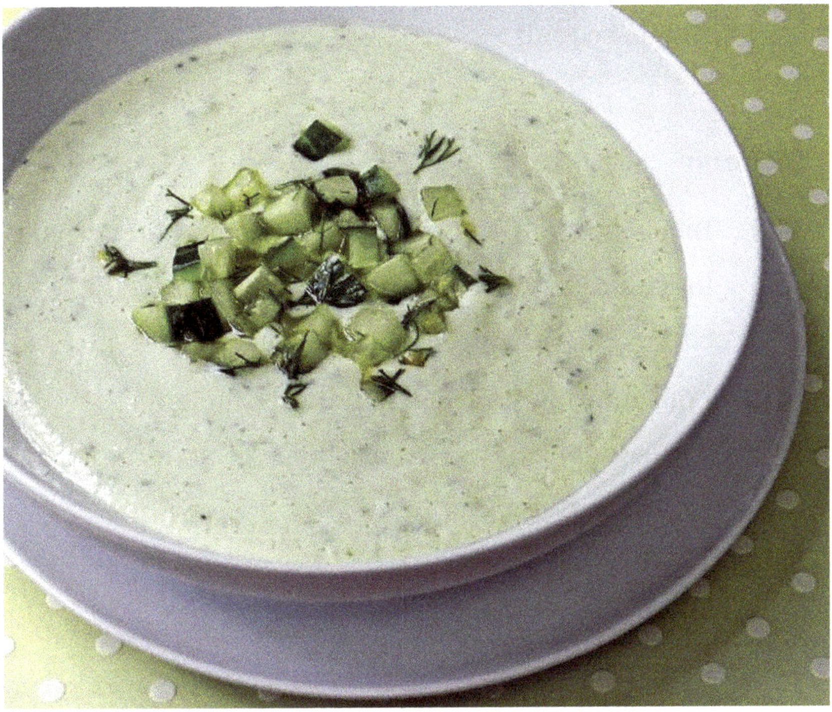

Preparation Time: 25 minutes

Cooking Time: 0 minute

Servings: 2

Ingredients:

- 1 cucumber, peeled
- ½ zucchini, peeled
- 1 tbsp. freshly squeezed lime juice

- 1 tbsp. fresh cilantro leaves
- garlic clove, crushed
- ¼ tsp. sea salt

Directions:

1. In a blender, blend together the cucumber, zucchini, lime juice, cilantro, garlic, and salt until well combined. Add more salt, if necessary.
2. Pour into 1 large or 2 small bowls and enjoy immediately, or refrigerate for 15 to 20 minutes to chill before serving.

Nutrition:

Calories: 254 Protein: 30g Fat: 8g

Coconut, Cilantro, and Jalapeño Soup

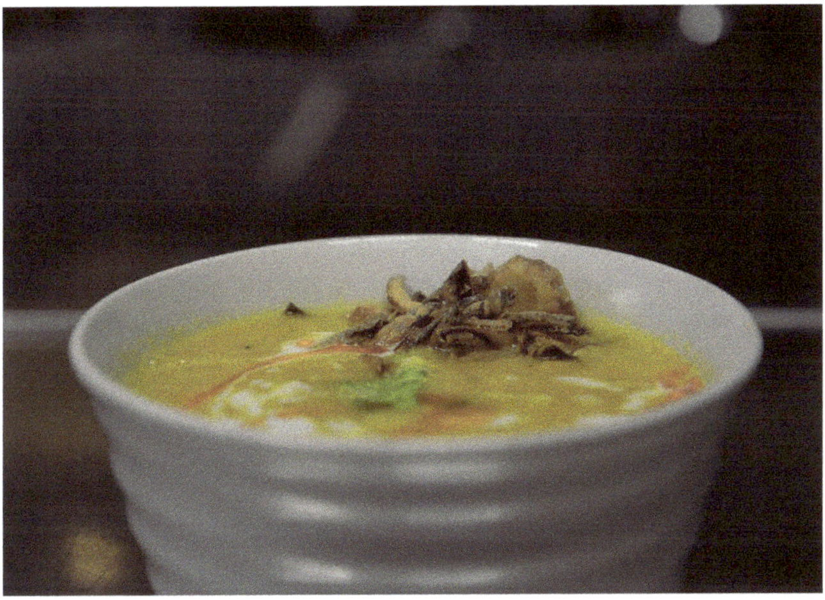

Preparation Time: 5 minutes

Cooking Time: 5 minutes

Servings: 2

Ingredients:

- tbsp. avocado oil
- ½ cup diced onions
- garlic cloves, crushed
- ¼ tsp. sea salt
- (13.5 oz.) can full-fat coconut milk

- 1 tbsp. freshly squeezed lime juice
- ½ to 1 jalapeño
- tbsp. fresh cilantro leaves

Directions:

1. Using a medium skillet over medium-high heat, heat up avocado oil. Sauté onion, garlic, and salt for 4minutes.
2. In a blender, blend together the coconut milk, lime juice, jalapeño, and cilantro with the onion mixture until creamy.
3. Pour into 1 large or 2 small bowls and enjoy.

Nutrition:

Calories: 159 Fat: 11g Protein: 37g

Spicy Watermelon Gazpacho

Preparation Time: 5 minutes

Cooking Time: 0 minute

Servings: 2

Ingredients:

- 2 cups cubed watermelon
- ¼ cup diced onion
- ¼ cup packed cilantro leaves
- ½ to 1 jalapeño
- 2 tbsp. freshly squeezed lime juice

Directions:

1. In a blender or food processor, pulse to combine the watermelon, onion, cilantro, jalapeño, and lime juice only long enough to break down the ingredients, leaving them very finely diced and taking care to not over process.
2. Pour into 1 large or 2 small bowls and enjoy.

Nutrition:

Calories: 207 Fat: 5g Protein: 36g

Roasted Carrot and Leek Soup

Preparation Time: 10 minutes

Cooking Time: 30 minutes

Servings: 2 to 4

Ingredients:

- 6 carrots
- cup chopped onion
- 1 fennel bulb, cubed
- garlic cloves, crushed
- 2 tbsp. avocado oil
- 1 tsp. sea salt
- tsp. freshly ground black pepper
- cups almond milk, plus more if desired

Directions:

1. Preheat the oven to 400°F. Line a baking sheet with parchment paper. Cut the carrots into thirds, and then cut each third in half. Transfer to a medium bowl.

2. Add the onion, fennel, garlic, and avocado oil, and toss to coat. Season with salt and pepper, and toss again.
3. Transfer the vegetables to the prepared baking sheet, and roast for30 minutes. Remove from the oven and allow the vegetables to cool.
4. In a high-speed blender, blend together the almond milk and roasted vegetables until creamy and smooth. Adjust the seasonings, if necessary, and add additional milk if you prefer a thinner consistency.
5. Pour into 2 large or 4 small bowls and enjoy.

Nutrition:

Calories: 220 Fiber: 15g Protein: 28g

Lemon Cauliflower & Pine Nuts

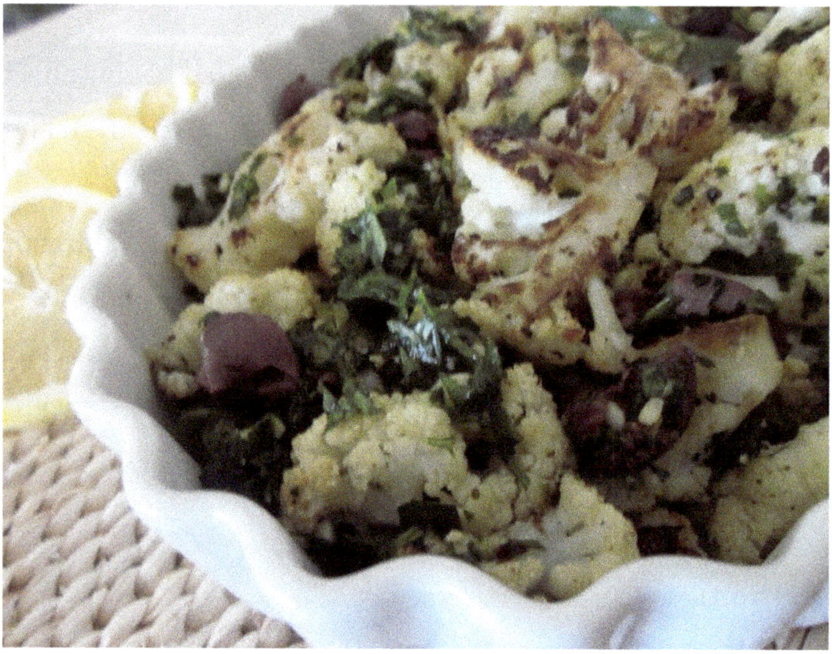

Preparation Time: 5 minutes

Cooking Time: 20 minutes

Servings: 4

Ingredients:

- 1 tsp. lemon zest
- ¼ tsp. sea salt
- (10 oz.) package cauliflower florets
- 2 tbsp. extra virgin olive oil

- tbsp. pine nuts
- 1 tbsp. parsley, fresh flat-leaf
- 1 ½ tsp. lemon juice
- ¼ tsp. fresh ground black pepper

Directions:

1. Preheat your oven to400°F.
2. In a large bowl, combine all of your ingredients. Then set onto a baking sheet.
3. Bake for 20 minutes, serve and enjoy!

Nutrition:

Calories: 60 Protein: 4g Fat: 0.1g

Beef Tenderloin & Avocado Cream

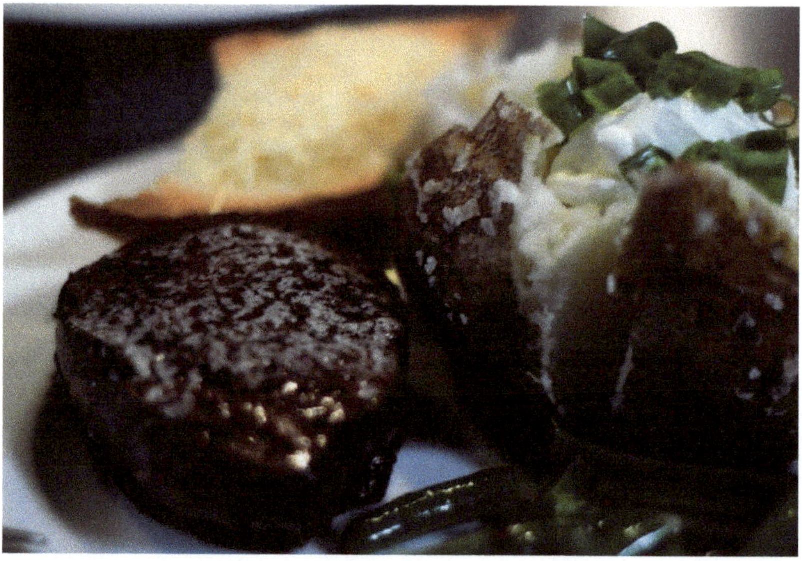

Preparation Time: 10 minutes

Cooking Time: 8 minutes

Servings: 2

Ingredients:

- tsp. Mustard
- (6 oz.) beefsteaks
- ¼ cup sour cream
- 2 tsp. lemon juice, fresh
- 1/3 avocado

- 1 tbsp. olive oil-slicked
- Sea salt along with fresh ground black pepper as needed

Directions:

1. Preheat your oven to450°F.
2. Sprinkle the beef steaks with some salt and pepper.
3. Mix the mustard and oil and spread the mixture over the meat.
4. Place the steaks into a skillet over medium-high heat for 3minutes.
5. Transfer the steaks to a baking sheet and place in the oven, then bake for 6minutes.
6. Blend the avocado with lemon juice and sour cream.
7. Serve steaks with avocado cream and enjoy!

Nutrition:

Calories: 205 Protein: 20g Fat: 15g

Salmon & Citrus Sauce

Preparation Time: 10 minutes

Cooking Time: 15 minutes

Servings: 2

Ingredients:

- ¾ lb. salmon fillets
- 1/3 cup fresh orange juice
- 1 tbsp. fresh lime juice
- 1 tbsp. fresh lemon juice
- 1 tbsp. honey
- 1 tbsp. olive oil
- 1 ½ tbsp. mustard
- Sea salt along with fresh ground black pepper as needed
- ¼ tsp. smoked paprika

Directions:

1. Sprinkle fillets with paprika, salt, and pepper. Then, cook in a skillet over medium-high heat for 5 minutes per side.

2. While fillets are cooking, mix the lemon, orange, lime juices, and honey, then add to a small saucepan. Add the mustard and stir to combine—Cook over low heat for 10minutes.
3. Add the salmon fillets to serving dishes, then pour the sauce over the fillets.
4. Serve and enjoy!

Nutrition:

Calories: 210 Protein: 20g Fat: 22g

Orange-Avocado Salad

Preparation Time: 10 minutes

Cooking Time: 0 minutes

Servings: 2

Ingredients:

- ½ tsp. arugula
- 1 avocado
- 1 navel orange
- 1 tbsp. fresh lime juice
- 1 tbsp. extra-virgin olive oil

Directions:

1. Mix your lime juice, arugula, and oil in a bowl.
2. Add the peeled and sectioned pieces of orange, then toss.
3. Add the diced avocado just before serving, then enjoy!

Nutrition:

Calories: 30 Protein: 2g Fat: 2g

Avocados with Walnut-Herb

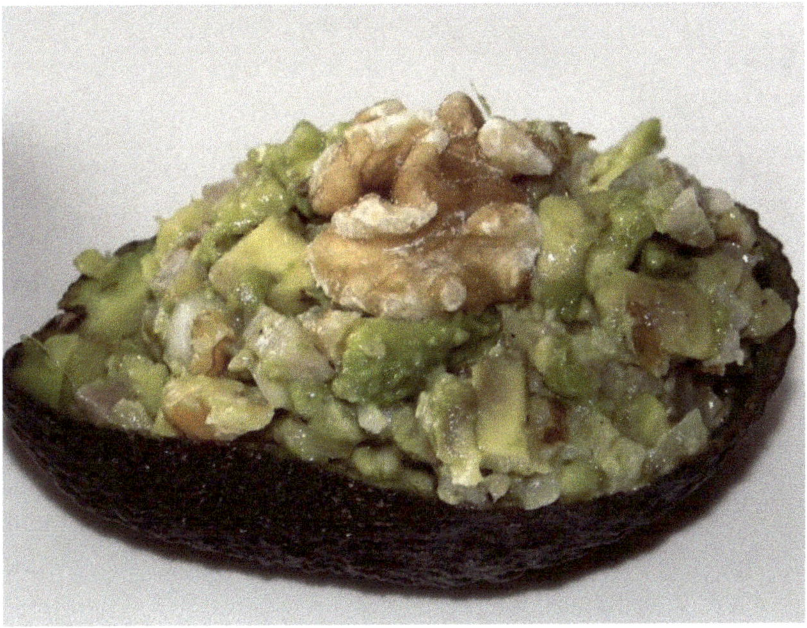

Preparation Time: 7 minutes

Cooking Time: 5 minutes

Servings: 2

Ingredients:

- 1 avocado
- ¼ cup walnuts
- 1 ½ tsp. virgin olive oil
- 1 ½ tsp. lemon juice (fresh)

- 1 tbsp. fresh basil
- sea salt and black pepper to taste

Directions:

1. Fry the chopped nuts for about 5 minutes over medium-low heat in a pan.
2. In a small bowl, mix the chopped basil, lemon juice, oil, sea salt, and pepper.
3. Slice avocado in half, then top slices with the walnut mixture, serve, and enjoy!

Nutrition:

Calories: 200 Protein: 2g Fat: 17g

Barbecue Brisket

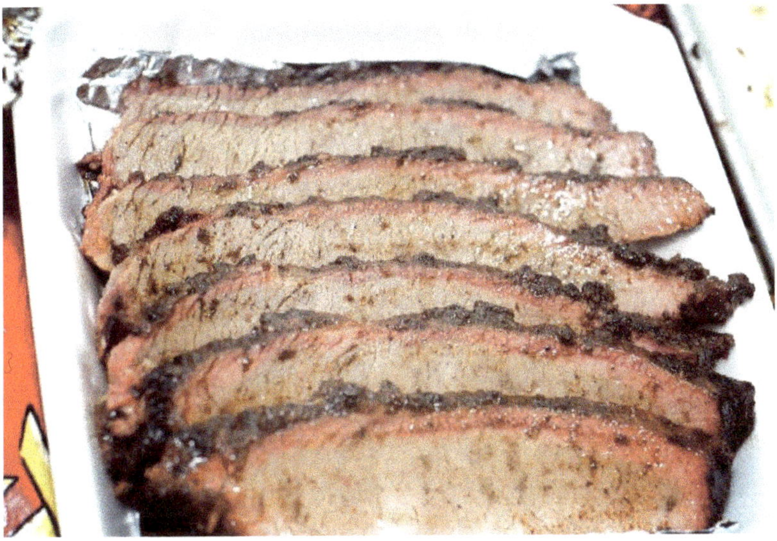

Preparation Time: 15 minutes

Cooking Time: 5 hours

Servings: 4

Ingredients:

- 1 cup beef broth
- 2 lb. beef brisket
- 1 sweet onion, diced
- ½ cup barbecue sauce
- ½ tbsp. steak seasoning

Directions:

1. Add the prepared onion to your slow cooker. Rub the trimmed brisket with seasoning.
2. Cut the brisket into pieces, and add to your slow cooker.
3. Pour the beef broth and barbecue sauce over the brisket.
4. Cook on low for 5 hours, slice brisket. Serve and enjoy!

Nutrition:

Calories: 188 Protein: 13g Fat: 8g

Broccoli & Hot Sauce

Preparation Time: 5 minutes

Cooking Time: 5 minutes

Servings: 4

Ingredients:

- 4 cups broccoli florets
- 1 tbsp. extra-virgin olive oil
- ½ tsp. hot sauce
- Sea salt along with black ground pepper as needed

Directions:

1. Arrange your broccoli in a steamer basket. Steam your broccoli for about 5 minutes or until tender.
2. Drizzle with the oil and sprinkle with hot sauce, sea salt, and black pepper. Serve and enjoy!

Nutrition:

Calories: 30 Protein: 4g Fat: 0.1g

Chicken Thighs

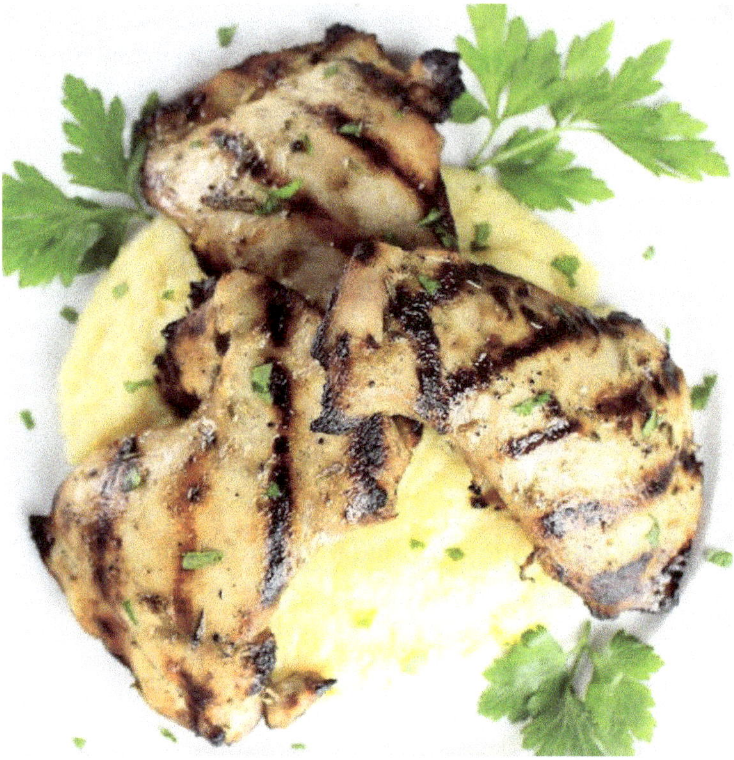

Preparation Time: 10 minutes

Cooking Time: 40 minutes

Servings: 4

Ingredients:

- 4 bone-in skinless chicken thighs
- ½ tsp. ginger

- tbsp. olive oil
- 2 tbsp. soy sauce
- ¼ tsp. dry mustard
- 1 garlic clove
- ¼ tsp. red pepper
- ¼ tsp. all-spice

Directions:

1. Preheat the oven to 400°F and sauté the minced garlic, ground allspice, ground ginger, crushed red pepper, and mustard in hot oil for 5 minutes. Remove from heat.
2. Whisk in soy sauce, then place the chicken thighs on a baking sheet. Add the garlic mixture over the chicken, and toss.

Nutrition:

Calories: 120 Protein: 8g Fat: 5g

Creamy Bell Pepper-Corn Salad & Seared Zucchini

Preparation Time: 10 minutes

Cooking Time: 20 minutes

Servings: 5

Ingredients:

- zucchinis
- ½ cup celery
- green bell pepper, sliced and seeded
- 1 dozen cherry tomatoes
- cups kernel corn
- 4 tbsp. sour cream
- ½ cup mayonnaise 2 tsp. sweetener
- sea salt along with ground black pepper as needed

Directions:

1. Cook your corn by following package instructions.
2. Mix the chopped celery, sliced bell pepper, whole cherry tomatoes, mayonnaise, sour cream, sweetener, salt, and pepper in a large salad bowl.

3. Heat a skillet over medium-high heat. Cook the zucchini sliced lengthwise for about 10 minutes. Turn occasionally, then add salt to zucchini.
4. Once zucchini is cooked, add it to the corn mixture.
5. You can serve this dish alongside your favorite meat dish!

Nutrition:

Calories: 100 Protein: 6g Fat: 3g

Sweet Potato, Kale, and White Bean Stew

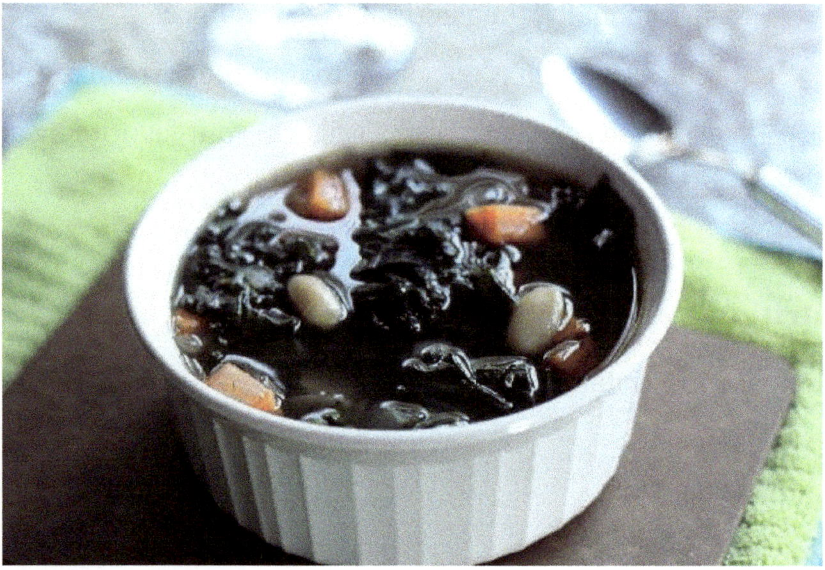

Preparation Time: 15 minutes

Cooking Time: 25 minutes

Servings: 4

Ingredients:

- 1 (15-ounce) can low-sodium cannellini beans, rinsed and drained, divided
- 1 tablespoon olive oil
- 1 medium onion, chopped
- 2 garlic cloves, minced

- 2 celery stalks, chopped
- 3 medium carrots, chopped
- 2 cups low-sodium vegetable broth
- 1 teaspoon apple cider vinegar
- 2 medium sweet potatoes (about 1¼ pounds)
- 2 cups chopped kale
- 1 cup shelled edamame
- ¼ cup quinoa
- 1 teaspoon dried thyme
- 1/2 teaspoon cayenne pepper
- 1/2 teaspoon salt
- ¼ teaspoon freshly ground black pepper

Direction:

1. Put half the beans into a blender and blend until smooth. Set aside.
2. In a large soup pot over medium heat, heat the oil. When the oil is shining, include the onion and garlic, and cook until the onion softens and the garlic is sweet, about 3 minutes.
3. Add the celery and carrots, and continue cooking until the vegetables soften, about 5 minutes.
4. Add the broth, vinegar, sweet potatoes, unblended beans, kale, edamame, and quinoa, and bring the

mixture to a boil. Reduce the heat and simmer until the vegetables soften, about 10 minutes.

5. Add the blended beans, thyme, cayenne, salt, and black pepper, increase the heat to medium-high, and bring the mixture to a boil. Reduce the heat and simmer, uncovered, until the flavors combine, about 5 minutes.
6. Into each of 4 containers, scoop 1¾ cups of stew.

Nutrition:

Calories: 373; total fat: 7g; saturated fat: 1g; protein: 15g; total carbs: 65g; fiber: 15g; sugar: 13g; sodium: 540mg

Slow Cooker Two-Bean Sloppy Joes

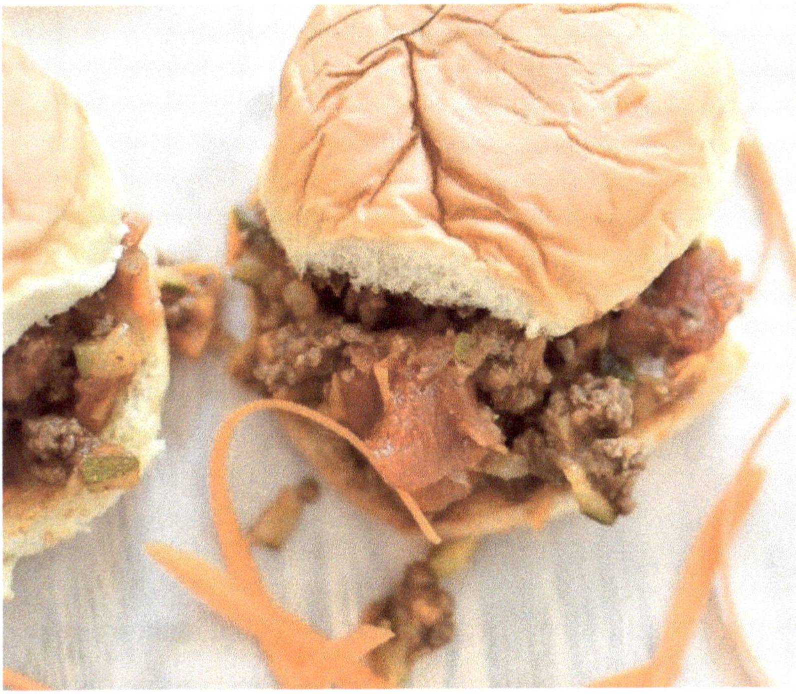

Preparation Time: 10 minutes

Cooking Time: 6 hours

Servings: 4

Ingredients:

- (15-ounce) can low-sodium black beans
- (15-ounce) can low-sodium pinto beans
- (15-ounce) can no-salt-added diced tomatoes

- medium green bell pepper, cored, seeded, and chopped
- 1 medium yellow onion, chopped
- ¼ cup low-sodium vegetable broth
- 2 garlic cloves, minced
- 2 servings (¼ cup) meal prep barbecue sauce or bottled barbecue sauce
- ¼ teaspoon salt
- ¼ teaspoon freshly ground black pepper
- 4 whole-wheat buns

Direction:

1. In a slow cooker, combine the black beans, pinto beans, diced tomatoes, bell pepper, onion, broth, garlic, meal prep barbecue sauce, salt, and black pepper.
2. Stir the ingredients, then cover and cook on low for 6 hours.
3. Into each of 4 containers, spoon 1¼ cups of sloppy sloppy joe mix.
4. Serve with 1 whole-wheat bun.
5. Storage: place airtight containers in the refrigerator for up to 1 week. To freeze, place freezer-safe containers in the freezer for up to 2 months. To

defrost, refrigerate overnight. To reheat individual portions, microwave uncovered on high for 2 to 21/2 minutes. Alternatively, reheat the entire dish in a saucepan on the stove top. Bring the sloppy joes to a boil, then reduce the heat and simmer until heated through, 10 to 15 minutes.

6. Serve with a whole-wheat bun.

Nutrition:

Calories: 392; total fat: 3g; saturated fat: 0g; protein: 17g; total carbs: 79g; fiber: 19g; sugar: 15g; sodium: 759mg

Lighter Eggplant Parmesan

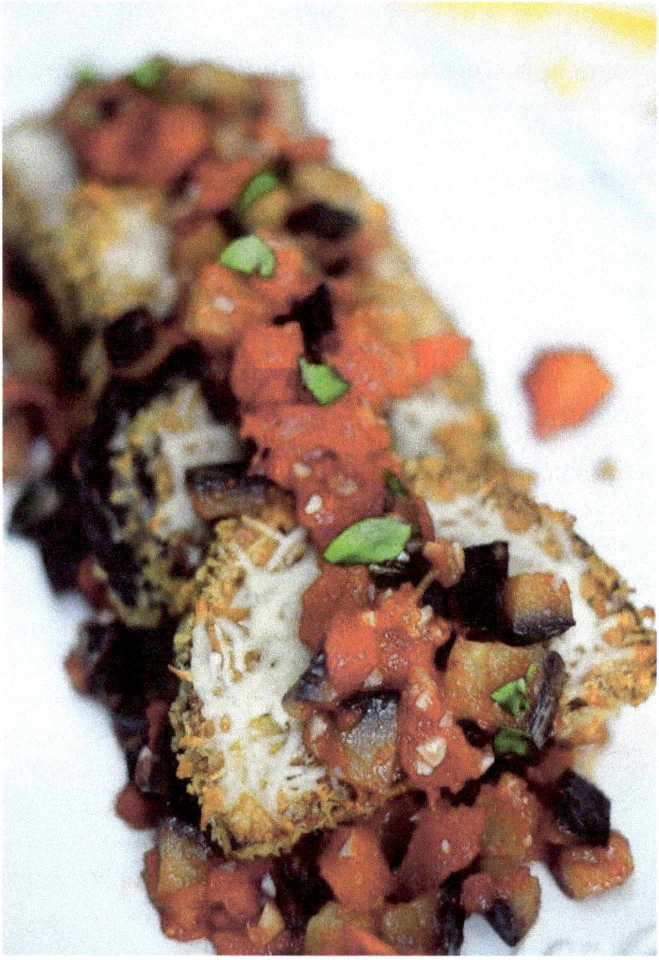

Preparation Time: 15 minutes

Cooking Time: 35 minutes

Servings: 4

Ingredients:

- Nonstick cooking spray
- 3 eggs, beaten, 1 tablespoon dried parsley
- 2 teaspoons ground oregano
- 1/8 teaspoon freshly ground black pepper
- 1 cup panko bread crumbs, preferably whole-wheat
- 1 large eggplant (about 2 pounds)
- 5 servings (21/2 cups) chunky tomato sauce or jarred low-sodium tomato sauce
- cup part-skim mozzarella cheese
- ¼ cup grated parmesan cheese

Direction:

1. Preheat the oven to 450f. Coat a baking sheet with cooking spray.
2. In a medium bowl, whisk together the eggs, parsley, oregano, and pepper.
3. Pour the panko into a separate medium bowl.
4. Slice the eggplant into ¼-inch-thick slices.
5. Dip each slice of eggplant into the egg mixture, shaking off the excess.
6. Then dredge both sides of the eggplant in the panko bread crumbs. Place the coated eggplant on the

prepared baking sheet, leaving a 1/2-inch space between each slice.

7. Bake for about 15 minutes until soft and golden brown. Remove from the oven and set aside to slightly cool.
8. Pour 1/2 cup of chunky tomato sauce on the bottom of an 8-by-15-inch baking dish. Using a spatula or the back of a spoon spread the tomato sauce evenly. Place half the slices of cooked eggplant, slightly overlapping, in the dish, and top with 1 cup of chunky tomato sauce, 1/2 cup of mozzarella and 2 tablespoons of grated parmesan. Repeat the layer, ending with the cheese.
9. Bake uncovered for 20 minutes until the cheese is bubbling and slightly browned.
10. Remove from the oven and allow cooling for 15 minutes before dividing the eggplant equally into 4 separate containers.

Nutrition:

Calories: 333; total fat: 14g; saturated fat: 6g; protein: 20g; total carbs: 35g; fiber: 11g; sugar: 15g

Coconut-Lentil Curry

Preparation Time: 15 minutes

Cooking Time: 35 minutes

Servings: 4

Ingredients:

- tablespoon olive oil
- medium yellow onion, chopped,
- 1 garlic clove, minced
- medium red bell pepper, diced
- (15-ounce) can green or brown lentils, rinsed and drained
- 2 medium sweet potatoes, washed, peeled, and cut into bite-size chunks (about 1¼ pounds) 1 (15-ounce) can no-salt-added diced tomatoes
- 2 tablespoons tomato paste
- 4 teaspoons curry powder
- 1/8 teaspoon ground cloves
- (15-ounce) can light coconut milk
- ¼ teaspoon salt
- 2 pieces whole-wheat naan bread, halved, or 4 slices crusty bread

Direction:

1. In a large saucepan over medium heat, heat the olive oil. When the oil is shimmering, add both the onion and garlic and cook until the onion softens and the garlic is sweet, for about 3 minutes.
2. Add the bell pepper and continue cooking until it softens, about 5 minutes more. Add the lentils, sweet potatoes, tomatoes, tomato paste, curry powder, and cloves, and bring the mixture to a boil. are softened, about 20 minutes.
3. Reduce the heat to medium-low, cover, and simmer until the potatoes
4. Add the coconut milk and salt, and return to a boil. Reduce the heat and simmer until the flavors combine, about 5 minutes.
5. Into each of 4 containers, spoon 2 cups of curry.
6. Enjoy each serving with half of a piece of naan bread or 1 slice of crusty bread.

Nutrition:

Calories: 559; total fat: 16g; saturated fat: 7g; protein: 16g; total carbs: 86g; fiber: 16g; sugar: 18g; sodium: 819mg

Stuffed Portobello with Cheese

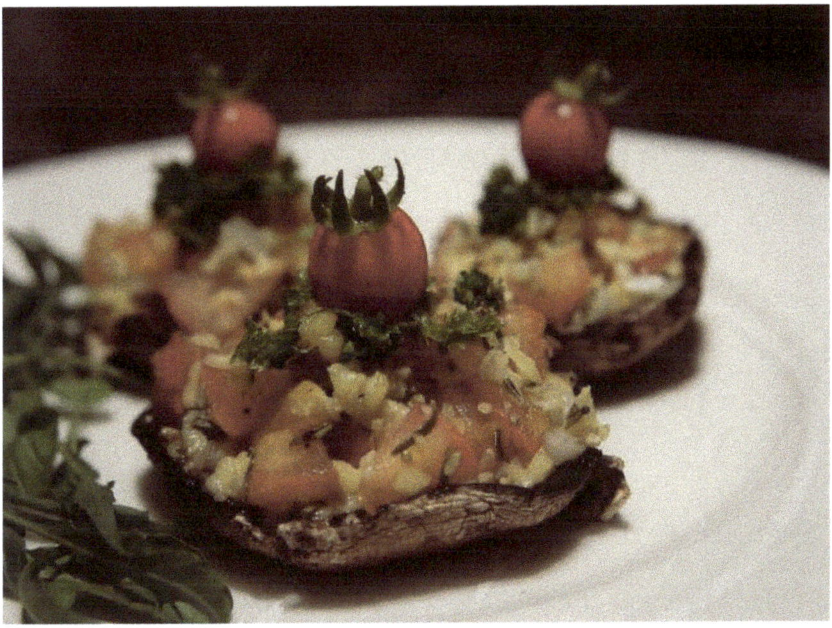

Preparation Time: 15 minutes

Cooking Time: 25 minutes

Servings: 4

Ingredients:

- 4 Portobello mushroom caps
- tablespoon olive oil
- 1/2 teaspoon salt, divided
- ¼ teaspoon freshly ground black pepper, divided

- cup baby spinach, chopped
- 11/2 cups part-skim ricotta cheese
- 1/2 cup part-skim shredded mozzarella cheese
- ¼ cup grated parmesan cheese
- garlic clove, minced
- tablespoon dried parsley
- 2 teaspoons dried oregano
- 4 teaspoons unseasoned bread crumbs, divided
- 4 servings (4 cups) roasted broccoli with shallots

Direction:

1. Preheat the oven to 375f. Line a baking sheet with aluminum foil.
2. Brush the mushroom caps with the olive oil, and sprinkle with ¼ teaspoon salt and 1/8 teaspoon pepper. Put the mushroom caps on the prepared baking sheet and bake until soft, about 12 minutes.
3. In a medium bowl, mix together the spinach, ricotta, mozzarella, parmesan, garlic, parsley, oregano, and the remaining ¼ teaspoon of salt and 1/8 teaspoon of pepper.
4. Spoon 1/2 cup of cheese mixture into each mushroom cap, and sprinkle each with 1 teaspoon of bread

crumbs. Return the mushrooms to the oven for an additional 8 to 10 minutes until warmed through.

5. Remove from the oven and allow the mushrooms to cool for about 10 minutes before placing each in an individual container.
6. Add 1 cup of roasted broccoli with shallots to each container.

Nutrition:

Calories: 419; total fat: 30g; saturated fat: 10g; protein: 23g; total carbs: 19g; fiber: 2g; sugar: 3g; sodium: 790mg

Lighter Shrimp Scampi

Preparation Time: 15 minutes

Cooking Time: 15 minutes

Servings: 4

Ingredients:

- 11/2 pounds large peeled and deveined shrimp
- ¼ teaspoon salt
- 1/8 teaspoon freshly ground black pepper
- 2 tablespoons olive oil
- shallot, chopped
- 2 garlic cloves, minced
- ¼ cup cooking white wine
- Juice of 1/2 lemon (1 tablespoon)
- 1/2 teaspoon sriracha
- 2 tablespoons unsalted butter, at room temperature
- ¼ cup chopped fresh parsley
- 4 servings (6 cups) zucchini noodles with lemon vinaigrette

Direction:

1. Season the shrimp with the salt and pepper. In a medium saucepan over medium heat, heat the oil. Add the shallot and garlic, and cook until the shallot softens and the garlic is fragrant, about 3 minutes.
2. Add the shrimp, cover, and cook until opaque, 2 to 3 minutes on each side.
3. Using a slotted spoon, transfer the shrimp to a large plate.
4. Add the wine, lemon juice, and sriracha to the saucepan, and stir to combine. Bring the mixture to a boil, then reduce the heat and simmer until the liquid is reduced by about half, 3 minutes.
5. Add the butter and stir until melted, about 3 minutes. Return the shrimp to the saucepan and toss to coat. Add the parsley and stir to combine.
6. Into each of 4 containers, place 11/2 cups of zucchini noodles with lemon vinaigrette, and top with ¾ cup of scampi.

Nutrition:

Calories: 364; total fat: 21g; saturated fat: 6g; protein: 37g; total carbs: 10g; fiber: 2g; sugar: 6g; sodium: 557mg

Maple-Mustard Salmon

Preparation Time: 10 minutes, plus 30 minutes marinating time

Cooking Time: 20 minutes

Servings: 4

Ingredients:

- Nonstick cooking spray
- 1/2 cup 100% maple syrup
- 2 tablespoons Dijon mustard
- ¼ teaspoon salt
- 4 (5-ounce) salmon fillets
- 4 servings (4 cups) roasted broccoli with shallots
- 4 servings (2 cups) parsleyed whole-wheat couscous

Direction:

1. Preheat the oven to 400f. Line a baking sheet with aluminum foil and coat with cooking spray.
2. In a medium bowl, whisk together the maple syrup, mustard, and salt until smooth.

3. Put the salmon fillets into the bowl and toss to coat. Cover and place in the refrigerator to marinate for at least 30 minutes and up to overnight.
4. Shake off excess marinade from the salmon fillets and place them on the prepared baking sheet, leaving a 1-inch space between each fillet. Discard the extra marinade.
5. Bake for about 20 minutes until the salmon is opaque and a thermometer inserted in the thickest part of a fillet reads 145f.
6. Into each of 4 resealable containers, place 1 salmon fillet, 1 cup of roasted broccoli with shallots, and 1/2 cup of parsleyed whole-wheat couscous.

Nutrition:

Calories: 601; total fat: 29g; saturated fat: 4g; protein: 36g; total carbs: 51g; fiber: 3g; sugar: 23g; sodium: 610mg

Milton Keynes UK
Ingram Content Group UK Ltd.
UKHW051923110124
435890UK00007B/51

9 781803 424842